It Isn't Common Sense

Interacting With People Who Have Memory Loss Due To Dementia

by

Jennifer Ghent-Fuller B.A. M.Sc.N.

Thoughtful Dementia Care ™

It Isn't Common Sense: Interacting With People Who Have Memory Loss Due To Dementia

By Jennifer Ghent-Fuller

Copyright 2013 by Thoughtful Dementia Care Inc.

Thoughtful Dementia Care ™

ISBN - 13: 978-1481995993

ISBN - 10: 1481995995

website: http://www.understanding-dementia-experience.com

Table of Contents

Introduction

People who live with a person with dementia, due to Alzheimer's disease or another similar progressive disease, experience a change in their previous pattern of interactions with that person. The person with dementia often shows a high anxiety level. This high anxiety level persists over much of their day, and as a result, they are irritable. Events occur that they do not expect to happen. They find themselves in situations that they cannot figure out and may feel that they cannot solve the dilemma of not knowing where they are or what is happening. People with dementia may develop a lack of trust in the people around them and a fear about what will happen next. With the ongoing accumulation of the changes in their abilities to comprehend and act, a person with dementia is less and less able to count on the world around them to be predictable and stable.

Years of working with people with dementia and their families and other carers have taught me that argument, impatience and anxiety are very often dominant in the social landscape of the family coping with dementia in one of its members. Dementia does not cause physical pain, however, it does cause emotional pain for the person who has it and also for everyone involved in their care. The approach outlined here has been successful in alleviating some of this emotional pain for many families, and it is hoped that it can be useful to others.

Relating to a person with dementia is not something people can do using their 'common sense.' What we consider to be 'common sense' is based on both members of a relationship having intact cognition. When short-term and long-term memory has been altered by disease, a person with dementia no longer has their former skill of using 'common sense,' and those around them need to alter their approach in how they relate and interact. People who are caring for someone with dementia need educational training to understand the interaction patterns that are suitable to use.

The brain is what we use to adapt our behaviour and responses to changes in our lives. A person with dementia has lost much of the ability to adapt. Understanding how the changes in the brain affect the way a person with dementia is able to think is the first step to knowing how to interact with them to alleviate their anxiety and help them stay calm. Changes in the way a person with dementia thinks, also result in changes in the ways they feel. To help the reader acquire a simple orientation to dementia an easily understood description has been provided, together with online search terms, designed to lead to the most relevant images.

"It Isn't Common Sense: Interacting With People Who Have Memory Loss Due To Dementia" is meant as further support for people who have read, or plan to read, "Thoughtful Dementia Care™: Understanding the Dementia Experience." "It Isn't Common Sense" addresses only the most fundamental changes in interaction patterns that are needed by carers of people with dementia. Reflective exercises are provided in order to help the carer build an understanding of the emotional context within which the person with dementia dwells, and to further deepen the carer's understanding of the dementia experience. This deep understanding is the ultimate guide to useful interaction with a person with dementia.

It is hoped that this guidebook will help those who are helping people with dementia, the carers, to develop the knowledge and skills to interact with a person with dementia, in order to create and maintain an emotional environment of trust and safety. This will help them to maintain a sense of security and enjoyment of life despite the enormous changes that are taking place in their ability to understand their world.

While we are all waiting for a future cure for Alzheimer's disease and other diseases causing dementia, what is needed in the meantime, by both the person with dementia and their carers, is a more peaceful journey through dementia. The presence of dementia in a family member leads to much grieving, tragedy, and physical and emotional hardship throughout the journey. If this journey is also laden with arguments, fights, accusations and recriminations, it adds to the grieving and makes the suffering that much worse.

A quick summary of interaction patterns that are helpful is available as a brochure: "How to Interact with a Person with Dementia," written in 2000. This brochure has been reproduced in its entirety at the end of the free ebook "Understanding the Dementia Experience," written in 2012. The latter has been expanded in the book "Thoughtful Dementia Care™." To locate these items, please visit http://www.understanding-dementia-experience.com.

1. The Feelings Caused by Forgetfulness

All of us are forgetful occasionally. It is a normal part of everyday life. When we are forgetful, it can cause changes in our emotional feelings. The following exercise will help you to understand the person with dementia who is forgetful and who recognizes that they are being forgetful. Their feelings will also be affected by being forgetful more than just occasionally. They are likely to be forgetful dozens, and even hundreds, of times per day.

If you have a friend that you can talk to as you work through the exercises in this book, that is a preferable way of completing it. However, if you are doing it on your own, please write your answers down so you can give yourself enough time to remember the details and the opportunity to think carefully.

Exercise. A. Describe the last time you forgot something. If you are on your own, write a brief note about the last time you forgot something.

_____

_____

B. Did your forgetfulness mean that you could no longer do what you had planned to do that day? Did it take more time for you do complete your work or activity?

_____

_____

C. What feelings did you experience during this event when you were forgetful? There is a list of feelings on page 38. Please consult it and write down two or three which closely describe some of the feelings you had on this occasion.

_____

_____

D. What were the reactions of other people?

Were they annoyed, angry or hurt? _____

Did they make fun of you? _____

Did they try to calm you down and say it didn't matter?

_____

E. How did the reactions of others make you feel? Please consult the list of feelings on page 38 and note whether there were any feelings added, by the reactions of others, to what you were already feeling about your forgetfulness.

_____

_____

F. If you felt badly when you were forgetful, what type of reaction by the other people would have been the best one to keep you from feeling worse?

_____

_____

Some people with dementia cannot recognize that they are forgetful because the area of the brain that permits them to have insight into their own abilities and behaviour is no longer functioning. Please read the section on Insight in the book "Thoughtful Dementia Care Care™: Understanding the Dementia Experience" for an explanation of the way insight may be affected by dementia.

It is normal for other people to think at the beginning that a person who is developing dementia is not doing things properly because they are unwilling, too lazy, too stubborn or unkind. It is very important to understand that people with dementia are not doing things properly because they no longer have the understanding, ability and 'common sense' that a properly functioning brain used to provide for them.

If, for example, you had a broken right arm and it was in a cast, how would you feel if someone yelled at you when you didn't use it the way you did before it was broken? Many people with dementia have someone yell at them or scold them because they are not doing things properly. If this is you, don't feel guilt, just continue reading.

Exercise. Think for a moment about a woman with dementia who starts out to do the dishes by filling the sink with water right up to the top. If any dish is put into the sink, or she puts her hand into the sink, the water will overflow onto the floor. Say this woman is your mother or your wife. You have had to clean up water off the floor many times in the few weeks since she started doing this.

A. How do you feel? _____

B. How are you speaking to her? _____

C. What are you communicating with your words? _____

_____

D. What are you communicating with your tone of voice?_____

_____

She knows that the sink needs to be full to do the dishes, but she is no longer able to remember how much water to put in the sink. Her disease has changed her ability to know things in the same way that she did in the past.

People who have their brain function intact can develop control over the emotions that they feel and the emotional reactions they let other people see. It is human nature to have a negative emotional reaction the first time that things go wrong. However, the carer in the situation described above, can decide not to get upset and angry, the next time this woman with dementia overflows the sink. Even though it makes a lot of work for them to clean up the water, they can remain calm and kind as they talk to the woman with dementia.

Remaining calm will also give them a better chance to think clearly about how to avoid the situation in the future. Perhaps they can suggest that she dries the dishes while they wash. Perhaps they can fill the sink for her and gently suggest that she doesn't need any more water. Figuring out what set of circumstances will make it easy for the person with dementia to participate in the tasks and activities as much as they are able to, while creating a situation where they are not causing big problems, or dangerous situations, is a trial and error process. The carer has to try one thing after another to see what will work, and then stick with that plan until the progression of the person's dementia causes a need to change the process again.

"Whose problem is it?" is a good question to ask yourself.

In the situation above, filling the sink too full is a problem for both the person with dementia and the carer. When the water spills on the floor, the woman and others in the household are in danger of slipping, falling, and injuring themselves; and, their home is in danger of sustaining water damage. Taking steps to encourage the woman to get out of the habit of filling the sink is a step toward safety.

By filling the sink too full, the woman has demonstrated that she has lost the ability to evaluate the appropriate level of water in the sink. Memory loss interferes with new learning. This means that trying to teach a person with dementia what the correct level of water in the sink should be, in the way that you would teach a child learning it for the first time, will not be successful. Helping her change her daily pattern to rely on someone else to fill the sink and giving her another job to help her continue to feel useful, will help to promote safety and a calm and secure emotional environment.

Consider a different situation. A fellow is sweeping the floor for many hours a day. He cannot use the dustpan effectively, so the dirt is getting moved around. He only sweeps one area of the house, not the whole house. He is absorbed in his task and seems to find fulfillment in what he is doing. His wife gets exasperated. She cannot see any value in working for so long without accomplishing anything. She frequently tells him to stop. When she tries to take the broom away from him, he pushes her away. She scolds him for pushing her.

Whose problem is this? The man is not harming the house, he is not in danger from his continued sweeping; in fact, it is good exercise. His wife is not in danger from his sweeping either. However, to her it doesn't make sense for him to sweep for so long without actually cleaning the floor. She has to vacuum anyway, and she has to wait to vacuum until he's done sweeping, so they don't run into each other. She is extremely upset because she can't get through to him, she can't get him to understand that what he is doing is useless activity.

This is an illustration of common sense not being useful. He is experiencing sweeping as something he wants and needs to do. He would have agreed with his wife before he developed dementia, but now he is doing his best to be active and useful, and he feels driven to sweep. He is no longer capable of evaluating his activity in the same 'common sense' way that his wife does. However, he still has the right to choose his activities as long as they are not impinging on his wife's right to physical safety.

This fellow is not capable of adapting to his wife's wishes. He is meeting his need to be active and to feel useful. His wife, however, is capable of adapting to his changing needs. She can realize that he is sweeping because he feels the need to do so, for whatever reason, which she may never understand. She can help him feel good by telling him what a good job he is doing. She can replace the broom when it wears out. She can help other people in the family understand that he is meeting his needs with his activity. She can change her thinking so she does not see her husband's sweeping as a problem, but rather, a useful activity that keeps him occupied and content.

His wife will be feeling grief and frustration that he is no longer fully participating in the care of their home and belongings in the way he did before the dementia. Carers often express this type of grief by scolding or showing their anger in other ways. Realizing that they are feeling grief and calming themselves down, allows carers to plan how they will interact with the person with dementia, and how they will get the household tasks done alone while they care for the person with dementia.

Carers who react with anger and scolding are not bad people. They are ordinary people having a very human reaction. However, it is important to get past this anger and not make it a permanent part of the family's journey through dementia. Staying calm will also decrease the work burden of caring, since they will not have to cope with returned anger and frustration from the person with dementia.

The grief is best dealt with by getting support from organizations (Alzheimer / dementia support organizations) that have support groups and counsellors available. If this is not an option, reading self-help books, joining professionally-run on-line support forums (the forums need to be refereed to avoid carers unintentionally hurting each other's feelings by being critical or insulting), or finding support in a religious or community group may be helpful.

2. Understanding the Basics of the Brain

Most people never think about their brain. They think of their head when they are getting a haircut, or when they have a headache, or when they are putting on a hat or make-up, without any thoughts about what structures are inside their head and how they function. We can't see changes from dementia on the outside of a person's body. Many family members have said that the brain disease only became real to them when they saw pictures of the resulting alterations in the brain.

The brain stores all the information about what we know and what we can do in every aspect of our lives. If there is damage to the brain caused by injury or disease, it changes what we can remember, the information available to us in everyday life, and how our body moves and functions. A basic understanding of how the brain is constructed and how it functions will assist you to comprehend why there are such enormous changes in the way a person with dementia thinks, acts, and feels.

Brain cells are long, with many projections that touch other brain cells. Brain cells interact with each other through electrical and chemical connections.

When you learn new information or new skills, you grow new brain cells and new projections between existing brain cells.

Go into a search engine on your computer, such as "Google" and search for:

brain cell image

You will find drawings of brain cells and photographs of brain cells that have been taken with high magnification. While you are looking at these images, think about how delicate and fragile the brain cells are and how marvellous it is that all these cells working together make us into the person that we are.

Now do a search for:

brain cell connections image

You will see how brain cells connect and communicate with each other by forming networks.

When you do something for the first time, your brain will figure out what to do by drawing on its learning from past situations. For example, if you are trying to find a store you have never been to before, you will need to know approximately where it is. When you get to the location, you will either recognize the sign by its shape and colour pattern or logo, or by the words written on the sign.

If you go back to that store within the next week or so, you will be able to recall how you got there, and find your way easily. If you keep going regularly, you will have no difficulty. Your brain cells have formed a new pathway of connections that is firmly established and will help you remember easily. If you go to the store once and then never go there again, or not for a few years, you may not remember how to find the store.

Think of walking across a field of grass for the first time. If you walk the same way a few more times, the grass will get flat. If you walk on it many times a day for a few months, the grass will wear off and you will have a path that has bare ground. In a similar way, the more you repeat an item you are trying to learn or a skill you are trying to acquire, the more firmly established the pathway in your brain becomes, and the more easily you remember it. The connections between the brain cells that you use for the activity you are learning become stronger and stronger until it is effortless for you to remember how to do that activity.

Various parts of the brain have different functions. To see what parts of the brain are involved in the various things people do, perform an online search for

brain lobe function image

There are connecting pathways between the various parts of the brain. So, if you process the image of a rose you are seeing with your occipital lobe, your parietal lobe and temporal lobe will help you name it and speak the word 'rose', and your frontal lobe will help you decide whether or not to buy it.

As you look at these images, think about what would happen if there were to be damage to the various parts of the brain due to dementia.

3. What Happens To The Brain When People Get Dementia?

People with dementia forget many things and change in many ways because they have a disease that is destroying their brain cells and the connections between their brain cells. Therefore all the information that is stored in the brain cells and made available by the connections between different brain cells, starts to be destroyed.

These changes are not visible to others. The person with dementia continues to look the same, and sometimes remembers and sometimes does things without making the same mistakes they made just the day before. Others around them need to understand that the person with dementia has no choice in how the disease affects them. Becoming familiar with what is happening inside the brains of people with dementia, will help those caring for them comprehend why the person with dementia changes.

If the disease is progressive, that is, if it gets worse as time goes on, then more and more brain cells and brain cell connections will be destroyed and more knowledge and ability will be lost.

The term "dementia" refers to the condition of a person who no longer has all their brain function because of a progressive disease. There are many diseases that cause a progressive decline in brain function.

Over half the people who have dementia have Alzheimer's disease. A person can also have more than one type of disease that is causing their brain tissue to deteriorate.

Go online again and do a search for:

Alzheimer's brain cell images

You will see drawings and images of a material, called plaque, which is laid down between brain cells and interferes with their function. The internal structure of the brain cell breaks down and broken down brain cells become clumped together into formations called tangles. These plaques and tangles allow someone looking at brain tissue under a microscope to identify the disease as Alzheimer's disease.

Normally, brain tissue is not examined when a person is alive because it is too dangerous to take a sample, since doing so may cause further damage and trauma to the brain.

As the brain cells are destroyed, the brain itself starts to shrink. This shrinkage is not usually visible on a brain scan in the early stage of the disease, but it depends on the type of scanning that is available. Some of the more sophisticated scans are available only to researchers, not to doctors trying to make a diagnosis. This will change as the technology develops and becomes more widely available.

There are other common diseases, besides Alzheimer's disease, which cause dementia. You will see that each disease looks slightly different under a microscope.

Do an online search for:

Lewy Body brain cell image

Lewy bodies are found in the brains of people with Lewy body disease, and also people with Parkinson's disease. Not everyone with Parkinson's disease develops dementia.

Now do another search, this time for:

Pick bodies images

Pick bodies appear in the brains of people with Pick's disease. This disease is also called Frontal Lobe Dementia or Frontotemporal Dementia.

No matter what disease develops in the brain, there is damage to brain cells and to the connections between brain cells. With each of these progressive diseases, the brain damage eventually affects the entire brain. The early symptoms are sometimes different. For example, typically the first sign of Alzheimer's disease is short-term memory loss, whereas the early sign of Pick's disease may be a person making judgements they would not ordinarily make. People with Lewy Body disease often have hallucinations as an early sign.

Another progressive brain disease is slightly different. Vascular Dementia refers to disease in the blood vessels of the brain caused by small strokes. Small strokes may not produce any symptoms at first, but the accumulation of many small strokes in the brain produces widespread damage. To see examples of the impact on the brain of vascular dementia, do an online search for

multi-infarct dementia image

A stroke may also be called a cerebrovascular accident (CVA) or an infarct. When strokes happen, there is an interruption in the flow of blood that brings nutrition and oxygen to some brain cells, which causes those brain cells to die.

If there is a stroke in a large vessel, it may be immediately fatal, or it may cause widespread damage to the brain, resulting in loss of movement and many functions, such as language.

The smallest blood vessels are called capillaries. They may provide nutrition and oxygen to only a small number of brain cells. When a stroke is this small, no-one, including the person who has the stroke, may notice it or may see any resulting symptoms. Vascular dementia results when there are hundreds of these small strokes and the damage accumulates until it is noticeable. Usually this disease keeps progressing until it, too, affects the whole brain.

It is important to realize that not all strokes progress to dementia. It is also important to note that strokes are mainly preventable.

Search for:

stroke risk factors and prevention

if you would like more information about preventing vascular dementia.

It is very important to note that the same health practices that prevent strokes also help to prevent heart attacks and help prevent or delay the onset of other diseases causing

13

dementia. If someone already has a disease, good health practices may slow the progression of their dementia.

Strokes may be caused by the bursting of a blood vessel, resulting in the blood leaking into the rest of the brain. This is also called a hemorrhage. Other strokes are caused by the blockage of a blood vessel.

Search for

stroke image

to see illustrations of the damage to blood vessels and the brain that result from strokes.

Alzheimer's disease, Lewy Body disease, Parkinson's disease with dementia, Pick's Disease and Vascular Dementia are the diseases that are the main causes of dementia in the population. There are many other diseases that cause dementia. For more information, search online for

other dementias

If a person has dementia, the functions of the brain are changed. Below is a partial list of brain functions in no specific order. You can see from this list how enormously dependent we are on our brains functioning well.

- sensory perception, thinking or thought processing, reasoning, logic, evaluation of social interaction, suppressing behaviours, planning, organizing, risk evaluation, situational analysis, judgement, remembering, comprehending, attention, language comprehension and speech, learning, problem-solving, decision-making, dreaming, sensory information processing, emotional control, object recognition, facial recognition, feeling emotions, voluntary movement, muscle coordination, sleeping, awaking, staying awake, regulation of internal body functions such as digestion, respiration, excretion, body temperature, secretion of hormones, sexuality, reaction to danger, self-control, mathematical calculation, self-awareness, and insight.

4. Is It Really Dementia?

As the disease causing the dementia becomes more widespread in the brain, the person with the dementia loses more functions.

Diseases causing dementia mainly affect people who are over sixty-five. It is rare for someone younger than fifty to develop dementia, but it does happen.

Our population is aging. This means that the portion of the population that is older is growing. We have a greater proportion of the population over sixty-five years of age, than at any time in human history. This is happening because we have better nutrition, we have systems where we live that provide clean water and sewage removal, and we also have better disease diagnosis and treatment. This is allowing more people to reach old age. Since the diseases causing dementia mainly occur in older people, we are seeing more instances than we have in the past. The incidence of disease causing dementia is increasing. So it has become more important to learn how to care for people with dementia and how to diagnose and prevent diseases causing dementia.

Diagnosis by a physician or nurse practitioner is completed by:

- 1. Doing general tests to be sure that there is no other illness or medical condition present that is causing the symptoms. For example, older people are more likely than younger adults to develop delirium as a result of commonly occurring illnesses. Since conditions causing delirium are often treatable, it is important to seek medical attention as soon as symptoms appear. Symptoms of conditions causing delirium are more likely to appear suddenly, over a few days, rather than developing slowly as the symptoms of dementia do, but sometimes delirium does develop slowly. People who already have dementia can also have a condition causing delirium that is causing them to have worse symptoms. For more information, do an online search for:

causes of delirium in the elderly

- 2. Listening to family members tell how the person has changed. If you need to communicate this to the doctor it helps to put it in writing. One good way to organize your thoughts is to use a list of the most common symptoms of dementia and write down examples of each of these symptoms that you are seeing in the person about whom you are concerned. To help yourself do this, search for:

warning signs of dementia

- 3. Doing paper and pencil tests to see how much the person can remember. These tests have been developed by testing thousands of people and looking back to see whether the scores accurately predicted whether a person had dementia. It is important to remember that a person with delirium is also likely to do badly on these tests. That is why a general medical examination, the first step listed here, and a medical history (which includes medication usage and changes) are vital parts of diagnosis. Screening for dementia with paper and pencil or online tests alone is not accurate or adequate. You need professional interpretation of the test and access to ongoing support through a professional if it proves necessary.

- 4. Observing the person over time to see if their condition worsens. Dementia is a progressive condition, and if the person stays stable for six months to a year without new or worsening symptoms, they are very unlikely to have a progressive disease. Single strokes can cause a deficit which does not change or which gets slowly better. Oxygen deprivation during a heart attack can cause similar one-time injuries, which do not progress. Lifestyle changes, which will lessen the chance of future strokes or heart attacks, are the best option to prevent further injury.

All four elements must be present in the diagnostic process in order to arrive at the best diagnosis possible. At this point, there is no simple blood test or other test that can determine whether a person has a disease causing dementia. Instead, it requires skilled assessment of multiple symptoms over a period of time. Physicians who are specialists in the medical conditions of older people are called geriatricians. If you are uncertain about the diagnosis that has been made, you may want to ask for a second opinion.

5. Memory Changes

Five types of memory will be discussed:

- Short-term memory
- Long-term memory
- Immediate or Working memory
- Procedural Memory
- Emotional Memory

Exercise: Fill in which type of memory you think you are using in the following situations:

1. Remembering what you ate most recently: _____

2. Remembering your childhood: _____

3. Remembering how you felt when you got a piece of good news: _____

4. Remembering how to type: _____

5. Remembering the most recent sum when you are adding a column of numbers:

_____

5A. The Implications of Short-Term Memory Loss for Interaction

Short Term Memory is used in many day-to-day tasks involved in working and in caring for ourselves and our homes. If the family members, or carers, understand the limitations of the person with dementia, which are caused by their short-term memory loss, they will be able to help them avoid situations that will be too stressful, and will be able to help them compensate for their memory loss for the tasks they are performing. This will increase the quality of life of both the person with dementia and their carers.

If someone asked you what you had been doing for the past 10 minutes, what memory process would you be using to answer that question?

If you answered "short-term memory", you would be correct. We use our short-term memories to recall the events of the past week or so, whether it was 3 days ago or 5 minutes ago, and remind ourselves what we will be doing over the next couple of days.

(Answers to questions above: 1. Short-term memory, 2. Long-term memory,

3. Emotional memory, 4. Procedural memory, 5. Immediate memory.)

Here is a list of everyday things you do that require using your short term memory:

- Remembering the content of a conversation for a few days;
- Remembering the beginning of the book that you are half-way through reading, or the plot and characters of the movie or television show you are watching;
- Performing a complex task such as making dinner or fixing a motorcycle: remembering what portion of the task we have already done, what comes next and moving from one part of the task to another without losing track of the timing of each step and its sequence;
- Keeping more than one task in our mind at a time, for example, when driving, we keep track of where we are going, which lane we are in, what other cars are close to us, the speed we are going, and possibly we are conversing or listening to the radio at the same time;
- Remembering what day it is;
- Remembering how much time has gone by during the day;
- Remembering specifically what we have done so far today.

Write down three things that you have done today for which you needed to use your short-term memory.

1. _____

_____

2. _____

_____

3. _____

_____

Here are some everyday tasks that require the use of short-term memory to complete:

- using the telephone
- shopping
- food preparation
- housekeeping
- laundry
- driving or arranging transportation
- managing medications
- hobbies

- participating in community responsibilities such as clubs
- financial management
- most tasks we do in a work day for employment

As an example, here are the short-term memory tasks that are required to use the telephone successfully:

- remembering who you were about to call
- remembering the phone number that you have just looked up (if you don't have it memorized)
- remembering which single number you just dialed (out of the ten which comprise the whole phone number)
- remembering why you are calling
- remembering what you have already said in the conversation and what the other person has said
- remembering that you have already made the phone call so you don't make the same call again

Have a talk with a person who has dementia about something that has happened in the past week or so.

The next day, bring the topic up again.

Does the person with dementia remember the previous day's conversation?

Do they add information to the content and recall things on their own or do they merely comment on what you are saying now?

If the person with dementia has not remembered the conversation, how do you think they feel when you tell them about it? Refer to the list of emotions on page 38. Choose three that you think the person with dementia may be feeling.

——————————— , ——————————— , ———————————

Now, choose three emotions that you felt when the person you were talking to did not remember the conversation that you needed them to remember. Feel free to write emotions that are not included in the list.

——————————— , ——————————— , ———————————

If you were to become angry with them for not remembering, what emotions would they likely feel?

——————————— , ——————————— , ———————————

Generally speaking, when a person no longer has their short-term memory, or when it is faulty some of the time:

- Most things that happen are a surprise since they don't remember they are about to happen

- Conversations cannot be continued later because they may not remember the initial conversation about the topic

- People live 'in the moment,' not remembering what has just happened or what is about to happen

- Things get lost, since they do not remember where they put them down

- Most learning becomes impossible since new information cannot be rehearsed

- Complicated tasks or hobbies are impossible as many of the steps require short-term memory skills in order to know what has been done and what step is next

- Reasoning, logic and decision-making are increasingly harder because all the factors that need to be considered at the same time can no longer be considered at once. Usually a person with dementia can keep only one thing in their mind at a time.

5.B. The Implications of Long-term Memory Loss for Interaction

Why do you need to understand the impact of long-term memory loss on the life of your family member with dementia and on your own life? We use our long-term memory to guide our activities throughout the day.

Examine some basic activities that you might do and identify whether you are using your long-term memory. For example, consider making yourself a cup of coffee. Here is a list of some of the things you need to keep in your mind in order to make yourself a pot of coffee and pour yourself a cup. The type of memory used for each item is in brackets.

You need to know:

- when you last had coffee (Short-term memory)

- whether you need to restrict your caffeine level (Long-term memory)

- whether you have had your limit of coffee for the day (Short-term memory)

- where the coffee cups are kept (Long-term memory)

- that water is needed to make coffee (Long-term memory)

- that ground coffee beans are needed to make coffee (Long-term memory)

- that water comes from the tap (Long-term memory)

- how to turn on the tap (Procedural memory)

- how to coordinate your muscles to turn on the tap and hold the pot under the tap at the same time (Procedural memory)

- how to fill the pot with water (Procedural memory)

- to stop filling the pot with water at the correct level (Long-term memory)
- that the ground coffee goes in a basket in the coffee maker (Long-term memory)
- that a filter goes in the basket first (Long-term memory)
- where the filters are kept (Long-term memory)
- that only one filter is used (Long-term memory)
- how to coordinate your muscles to get only one filter out of the box (Procedural memory)
- how to correctly put the filter into the basket (Procedural memory)
- where the coffee is stored (Long-term memory)
- how much ground coffee you need to put into the basket (Long-term memory)
- whether you scoop out the coffee with a scoop or a spoon (Long-term memory)
- how to coordinate your muscles to put the coffee into the filter in the basket without spilling (Procedural memory)
- how to count the number of scoops to put into the basket (Short-term memory)
- that you have already put the ground coffee into the basket (Short-term memory)
- where the basket fits into the coffee maker (Long-term memory)
- how to lift the basket out and slide it back into place (Procedural memory)
- that the coffee maker needs to be plugged in (Long-term memory)
- that the coffee maker needs to be turned on with a switch to start brewing (Long-term memory)
- how to put the switch in the ON postion (Procedural memory)
- that you are in the middle of brewing a pot of coffee (Short-term memory)
- the sound made by the coffee maker while it's brewing (Long-term memory)
- that when the sound of brewing stops, and the coffee pot is full, the coffee is finished (Long-term memory)
- when to turn off the coffee maker (Long-term memory)
- how to recognize a cup (Long-term memory)
- where the cups are kept (Long-term memory)
- how to get the cup out of the cupboard and put it on the counter (Procedural memory)
- how to pick up the coffee pot by the handle properly so you don't burn yourself (Procedural memory)
- how to coordinate your muscles to pour the coffee into the cup (Procedural memory)
- to stop pouring coffee when you have enough in the cup (Long-term memory)

Our brains store an enormous amount of information, which we normally have access to without trying, in order to complete our everyday activities. However, if an area of knowledge is missing and the person cannot recognize a cup, know that a filter is needed, or no longer knows any one of the other items listed above, the person can no longer make a pot of coffee and pour themselves a cup.

Knowing that there may be only one or two steps unavailable to the person with dementia, you may be able to help them by assisting them to complete that step. If they are participating in making the coffee, and contributing as much as they can to the process, they will have higher self-esteem and feel that they are contributing in a useful way to looking after themselves and you.

It takes longer to help the person with dementia to perform a task such as making a pot of coffee, than it would to just do it yourself. The pace of your lives needs to slow down, at least when you are engaged in helping the person with dementia. If you are trying to move quickly, you will start to feel frustrated, and the person with dementia will sense your frustration and is likely to become anxious or upset in some way. Trying to urge the person with dementia to go faster than they are able to may cause them to become frustrated, anxious and upset.

When you are assisting a person with dementia to do any activities, it is most helpful to keep the mood upbeat and to have fun. This will be more pleasant for both of you. Also, if you become frustrated and begin to nag or scold, the person with dementia is more likely to resist your suggestions, and the whole activity will slow down or stop.

Pretend that you have dementia and you are sitting in your living-room. Suddenly a stranger walks into the room and starts talking to you as if you know them and you know what they are talking about. You don't know how they got into the house.

Please go to the sheet of emotions (pg. 38) and pick three that you might be feeling:

_____ , _____ , _____

Now, assume that the person who came into the living room is your spouse. They realize that you do not recognize them. How are they likely to be feeling?

_____ , _____ , _____

This type of event happens frequently to people with dementia due to Alzheimer's disease. Commonly, their long-term memories are erased backwards in time. The memories they have made most recently are erased first. As their disease progresses, they are only able to remember their early life. They may recognize a picture of their spouse when they were first married, without recognizing the same person as they appear at present.

The person with dementia has no choice about what they remember or what they have forgotten: no amount of convincing or arguing will enable them to retrieve the memories they have lost. However, even though they may not be able to name the person who is with them, this does not mean that they cannot feel comfortable with the person, and have a sense of belonging together. The pattern of interaction helps to establish this comfort level.

The person with dementia can continue to establish some new procedural memories. If the procedure of interaction is always kind, calm, accepting and slow, the person with dementia can feel confident and relaxed. Even if they are not able to name their spouse and state how they are related, they will be pleased to see them enter the room, and can be cooperative in the events of daily life since they feel secure.

Just for practise, write down three things that you would need to know in order to put clean sheets on your bed. Remember to list only the things that you have known for years.

1. _____

2. _____

3. _____

Now, think through this exercise to examine the emotions of a person with dementia. Pretend you are changing the sheets on your double bed.

You remember where the sheets are kept. You open the door to the cupboard. You see blue, white and green sheets. You forget that the green sheets are for a single bed. You try to put the green sheets on your bed and they don't fit. You can't do it. You have to start over again with the other sheets. This time, you try the white sheets. They are for a single bed too, and you can't get them on the bed.

Please look at the list of emotions on page 38. Pick two emotions from the list that you might be feeling right now.

1. _____

2. _____

Now, imagine that someone you live with comes into the room at this instant. There are three sets of sheets unfolded around the room – the ones you took off the bed, and the two that didn't fit. The person begins to look angry with you and yells at you. Does this change how you are feeling? Please look at the list of emotions again and identify how you might feel right now.

_____ / _____ / _____

Carers need to become experts in using patience and staying calm when they are interacting with a person with dementia. The person with dementia can make new procedural memories. It is important that the procedural memory they have when they see their carer is "this will be a pleasant time, this is a person who is nice to me."

5. C. Immediate Memory

The immediate or working memory continues to function for longer than the short-term memory in dementia of the Alzheimer's type. This is the type of memory that you use to keep track of a running total as you add a series of numbers, or count cups of flour you are adding to a recipe. Perhaps you can relate to having someone coming in and interrupting you. You lose your count and have to start all over again. This is also the memory that helps you keep track of a conversation. You are able to respond each time the other person says something. If you are interrupted, you may not remember what you had planned to say next. "Now, what was I saying?" is a common thing that is said when this happens. As soon as you are reminded, the memory comes back in a rush and you are able to continue.

A few pages ago, you were asked to analyze a conversation with a person with dementia and to answer the question: "Do they add information to the content and recall things on their own or do they merely comment on what you are saying now?" A person with some short-term memory loss, but whose working immediate memory is still available, will be able to add information to the content and recall other items they can remember which are pertinent to the conversation. A person without a working immediate memory is liable to comment only briefly with such responses as "Oh, yeah", "Un-Huh", "Oh, really", and so on.

However, their ability to converse also depends on what memories you are asking them to recall. If you are having a conversation about how well your daughter played basketball last week, you would be expecting them to recall something that happened recently, and in order to talk about it, they would have to also have a functioning short-term memory. If their short-term memory is not good, they will have very little to add to the conversation as their short-term memory has not allowed them to retain the information from the previous week.

If, instead, you are talking to them about something they did in their own childhood, for example whether they had a pet when they were small, they may still have many of those older long-term memories intact and will be able to give you information about their pet and how they used to play with it. They will be able to use their immediate memory to respond to what you are saying. This will be a more successful conversation.

Exercise. Try having a conversation with a person with dementia. Chose a topic that demands they use their short-term memory.

Now, have another conversation and chose a topic that lets them use the long-term memories that are still available to them. Note whether there is any difference in the degree to which they are engaged in the conversation. Are they talking in an animated way that shows they are enjoying themselves?

There are a couple of things to remember. As humans, we thrive on social contact such as conversations or sitting together as companions and enjoying something. It is usually the process of having a conversation, not the content of that conversation, which is important when it comes to interacting with a person with dementia. Conversing with them helps them feel that they are important and loved. They will still feel this way even if you have the same conversation over again on different days. With a short-term memory loss, they may not remember that you have talked about the same topic on many occasions. This depends, of-course, on how much short-term memory they retain.

Even though they have a lot of long-term memories, they may not be absolutely accurate in how they remember an event, or when something happened or to whom it happened. If you correct them, or scold them for not getting it right, you will change the process from something pleasant and enjoyable to something that creates negative feelings for you both.

Exercise. Try sitting to watch a TV drama with a person with short-term memory loss. Do they enjoy the show, or are they impatient and bored?

Although most people with short-term memory loss do not enjoy dramas because they are unable to keep track of the plot, some people do enjoy such shows if they are very familiar with them from their past. Even if they have an intact immediate memory, it is not sufficient to track an hour or half-hour long drama. Usually, watching something that does not require a good short-term memory is more successful. Many things can be found on the internet and played on the TV, such as a fire in the fireplace, or a nature film, or, sometimes a sports game works. A little experimenting about what is enjoyable for both of you can pay off in treasured time to relax together in a companionable way. Often, people with dementia are able to use their immediate memory to answer questions on game shows, or to complete a crossword puzzle. These activities permit thinking about only one thing at a time in the immediate present.

Understanding whether your interaction is demanding whether the person with dementia needs to use their short-term memory, their long-term memory and/or their immediate memory will help you plan for positive interactions which help them stay calm and relaxed and feeling secure. If someone other than yourself is spending time with the person with dementia, it will help if you set some guidelines about what activities and types of interaction are successful.

5.D. Procedural Memory

Typically, a person's procedural memory is available to them longer than the short-term memory in dementia of the Alzheimer's type. However, there are two patterns that seem contradictory. At the same time that a person is losing some of their procedural memories, they continue to be able to form new memories of some procedures. These memories are formed in a different way than memorizing new facts with repetition in the short-term memory. Procedural memories are formed when a person performs the same actions, or has the same experiences over and over again. An example of this would be a person with advanced dementia who lives in a nursing home. The new procedures that can be learned by a person with dementia are simple, one-step procedures. They may have forgotten the procedure of how to dress themselves, which requires multiple skills and an intact long-term and short-term memory. However over many weeks, they may learn new procedures, which require a single skill, such walking from their room to the dining room or to their favourite chair.

Exercise. In order to acquaint yourself with the workings of the procedural memory, please try a couple of exercises.

Think of a time when you drove a car that was unfamiliar to you. If you needed to drive in reverse, did your hand go automatically to the location of the hand gear in the old car? This is your procedural memory at work. In order for you to place your hand in the right position to change gears in the new car, you will have to look for the gear shift, or correct yourself a few times until your brain forms a pathway of new connections between cells. Then, you will be able to do it without looking, and without consciously thinking about being in a different car.

Simple procedures are the easiest ones for the person with dementia to continue doing as activities. Examples of this are raking leaves, drying dishes, sweeping or dusting. However, the person with dementia may perform a simplified version of even these one-step tasks. The person who is raking leaves may not know where to put the pile. The person drying dishes may not know how to put them away in the cupboard.

Even simple procedures often have a number of steps and smaller procedures that, when combined, form one task. Consider brushing your teeth. There are many steps - picking up the toothbrush, turning on the water, getting out the toothpaste, knowing how to change the angle of your hand and fingers to brush the front and back of all your teeth, and, rinsing your mouth. Usually, if a person stops doing a particular procedure, they need help with it from that time on. Because of the progressive nature of dementia, they may go through a period of not being able to do something one day, but doing it without any effort the next. This may go on for weeks until they finally stop being able to do it altogether. However, it is important to watch what is interfering with the completion of the task. For example, a person with dementia may not remember how a flip top toothpaste tube works, but they may still retain the ability to open a toothpaste tube that needs to have the lid unscrewed. Replacing the toothpaste tube with one they know how to manage may allow them to continue brushing their own teeth for many months.

Exercise. Think about how would you feel if one of your family members followed you into the bathroom, put toothpaste on your toothbrush and started brushing your teeth? This is not something that you are used to and you are very surprised. You'd likely feel strange and very uncomfortable.

A person with dementia would feel the same way. If there is someone without dementia in the family, who cannot use their hands for some reason, they would understand why another person is brushing their teeth. However, the person with dementia may not remember that they have not been brushing their teeth, even if they have been told this information many times. They need to be gently assisted to accept a new way of doing things, without ever having the possibility of understanding why it is necessary.

Getting a person with dementia used to any new way of doing things needs to be done slowly, with "baby steps." If you notice that they are having trouble successfully brushing their teeth, you can take the first step of getting them used to you being in the bathroom by following them there, chatting through the door, then staying in the bathroom, brushing your teeth at the same time beside them, putting the toothpaste on their brush, offering to help, and finally offering to give them a hand quietly and calmly and with a smile. This process of gradually encroaching on their privacy and taking over a job that they have always done themselves may take many days or longer. If you try to rush and do it before they are ready, they may resist your attempts and misinterpret what your intentions are. They may even feel that you are trying to harm them. Even though it takes a long time, it is worthwhile to avoid misunderstandings and anger, as this can lead to a person with dementia becoming resistant to accepting help.

The manner in which you offer help is also important. If you are rushed and trying to get a person with dementia to hurry, you are likely to be giving them demanding instructions and doing so repeatedly. If you can't get done what you expect to do, you may have to stop and evaluate your situation, rather than continuing and causing the both of you to feel stress.

What can you do to avoid having to rush? Starting to get ready earlier is one option. Additionally, reviewing what you are doing to make sure all of it is essential is helpful. For example, if your family member has always put on "good" clothes to go to medical appointments, is that still necessary? Will it do any harm to take Mom in her T-Shirt and sweat pants, rather than spend an hour or two helping her to change clothes? Ask for some help. For example, if Dad now needs to take pills six times during the day, ask the doctor to discontinue anything that is not essential and schedule them so you are helping with medications only once or twice a day. In other words, pare the list of all tasks down to only those that must be done, and then take as many short cuts as possible to eliminate any unnecessary steps.

Exercise. Think of yourself going into a grocery store. You cannot find the coffee. You look up all the aisles twice. Finally, you find a clerk and ask. The clerk is grumpy and angrily points to the aisle before leaving. Now, think of the emotions you would be feeling. Would you want to go to that store or talk to that clerk again? A person with dementia would have similar feelings if they were treated this way. Before they had dementia, they may have been understanding if a family member was grumpy, knowing they had a lot to do quickly. However, after the onset of dementia, it is difficult for that person to keep more than one thing in their mind. They will know that the person who is angry with them but not be able to integrate an understanding or empathy with the angry family member.

The manner you use to help a person with dementia through their daily routines actually becomes part of the procedure. While it may be difficult to plant a smile on your face and take a light-hearted and joking approach, it is very important to try. It is hard on both of you if there are constant arguments. The aim is to help the person with dementia gradually form an understanding that the new procedure of being helped with their personal care is not unpleasant, and is actually fun. The person with dementia cannot change the fact that they are having trouble with daily tasks, that it takes them longer to do everything and that they misinterpret peoples' intentions. They also have difficulty understanding that you are in a hurry and if you give them lots of information about what other responsibilities you have besides their care, they are likely to stop what they are doing in order to try to understand what you are saying. This slows things down even more. People with dementia do best when they have one thing in their mind and are gently and pleasantly kept on track.

Exercise. Imagine you have moved all the plates in your cupboard to a different place in the kitchen. How long would it take for you to stop going to the wrong cupboard to get a plate?

You would eventually be able to learn where the new places are for things, even if you completely re-arranged your kitchen. The person with dementia may find a change very overwhelming and it may stop them from being able to function in the kitchen. Many people have noticed that a person with dementia can make a simple meal in their own kitchen, but if they are at someone else's home, they are not able to do the same task.

In order to support a person with dementia, it is helpful to keep them in familiar surroundings for as long as possible. They use their retained procedural memories to find the things that they need to use. This is also true of finding the rooms in their home. If people with dementia visit in someone else's home, they are likely to repeatedly need help finding the bathroom or the bedroom, or navigating around the neighbourhood, even though they don't need that type of help in their own home. Their procedural memories are strongest for the home with which they are most familiar.

Most household tasks require a person to use many different types of memory in order to complete them. As an example, here are some of the things you need to remember in order to do a load of laundry.

Long-term memory: Where is the washing machine located? How do you load the washing machine? Where do you put the soap? How much soap do you use?

Short-term memory: When was the last time you did a load of washing? Did you check the pockets? When did you put the wash on today? Did you remember to add soap? Have you put the clothes in the dryer? Have you finished the wash and put the clean clothes away?

Procedural memory: Remembering how and being able to coordinate the movements to: put the clothes in the washing machine; set the dials on the washing machine; open the laundry soap, measure and pour the correct amount of soap; place the soap in the correct place; open the washer and place the clothes in the dryer; setting the dial on the dryer; removing the clothes from the dryer and performing all the movements to fold and hang up the clean clothes away.

You also use your judgement (Are your clothes dirty? Are there enough clothes for a load of wash? Do you have to separate colours or fabrics for this load of wash?) and insight (Did you wash the clothes adequately to get them clean? Did it take you about the right amount of time to get the wash done? Was your memory adequate to get the clothes out of the washer and dryer on time?). (For a more complete discussion on changes in judgement and insight, please see the sections entitled "Insight" and "Judgement" in "Thoughtful Dementia Care ™: Understanding the Dementia Experience.)

5.E. Emotional Memory

Having dementia causes great emotional turmoil. With other illnesses, we can work on rationalizing and adjusting to our new state of health or lack of good health. We can plan our future and enact our plans. However, we use our brain to do that rationalizing, adjusting, planning and enacting. When the brain is affected by disease, emotional adjustment to health changes is more difficult and, with dementia, eventually impossible to do alone.

Emotional memories that have been long buried, or rationalized away in the past, can become dominant and cause emotional turmoil in the present. People who suddenly become fearful of dogs, for example, may have been bitten as children, and with the dementia can no longer control the outward expression of their emotional reaction of fear and annoyance. Graver still, are the emotional scars that some people carry from suffering physical violence or emotional or psychological abuse in the past.

Others, who share the life of the person with dementia, can have a powerful effect on their ability to adjust emotionally by how they treat them, how they interact with them and how they are present for them throughout their terminal illness, their dying process.

Similar to the pattern of procedural memories, emotional memories that have been made in the past can be lost, however new emotional memories can also be made after the onset of dementia. When our brain forms an emotional memory, it does so without the need to practice, in contrast to memorizing something through repetition in the short-term memory.

Emotion is all-important in dementia. Losing memories and abilities creates an enormous amount of anxiety. In fact, people with dementia are so fearful sometimes of being alone that they will follow their main carer everywhere (like a shadow, hence "shadowing"). Even if their carer is gone for just a minute out of sight, they will be upset and ask where they were.

If you can't figure out the meaning of what the person with dementia is trying to communicate, try to understand the emotion they are feeling. Responding to their emotion in an appropriate way may be what they need. If they are laughing, laugh with them. If they are upset, give them comfort.

Showing your frustration will make a person with dementia more anxious. If you try to convince them that they don't need to be upset, your emotional communication to them will be lack of acceptance, anxiety, intolerance and impatience. A person with dementia may not be able to understand, remember, or rationalize the words you are saying, but they will understand the emotions you are choosing to communicate to them.

Try for emotional calmness and contentment as a form of emotional palliation.

If you do show frustration and anger, which is only to be expected now and then with the difficulties you face, as soon as you calm down and get a grip on things again, go to the person with dementia, apologize briefly and engage in a fun, light-hearted and warm communication about anything at all.

Exercise. Think of a situation in which you usually lose your temper.

Practice in your mind how you will have a different reaction the next time the situation recurs. Start by planning to have no reaction until you can think the situation through. You can withdraw temporarily, for example by saying that you forgot to do something in another room, and then leave the room without further comment, or say "Just a minute," if the person calls after you.

Understand what it is about the situation that makes you angry. Try to adjust how you think when this situation occurs.

Act out your modified response. Don't be discouraged if this takes you many times to revise your own emotional behaviour.

6. Interaction Patterns

6. A. Interaction that Accommodates Short-term Memory Loss

- *Answer repeated questions as if it's the first time they've been asked*

WHY ➔ Loss of the short-term memory does not allow the person to remember that they've already asked the question. If you tell them they have already asked the question, they are likely to become anxious or withdraw from conversation because they feel humiliation. Anxiety may increase the frequency with which they repeat the question.

- *If they forget, be gracious.*

WHY ➔ If you smile and stay calm, you will decrease the stress that both you and the person with dementia experience.

- *Give casual reminders about who you are.*

WHY ➔ Even though you may have reminded a person with dementia who you are even a few minutes ago, you may notice them looking at you with puzzlement or they may directly ask you who you are. People with severe short-term memory loss can keep only one thing in their mind at a time. As soon as they think about somebody else, they are distracted and the information about who you are disappears and is no longer available to them. They suddenly find themselves standing next to a stranger and become anxious and will demand an explanation.

You will remember that this happens repeatedly, however, they may not. Answers that refer to the current, concrete activity (for example, "I am helping you make breakfast") may provoke less anxiety than answers that force them to acknowledge how much they don't know (for example, "I live here.") Finding the type of answer that provides the greatest sense of security for the person with dementia requires trial and error; trying one approach after another until you find what is acceptable to the person with dementia. There is no general rule. Every person with dementia is different, and, the approach needed changes over time as their understanding alters because of the progression of disease in their brain.

You will be able to feel less frustrated and stressed if you actively establish what type of response is most successful, and stick to it until it needs to be changed. Success is decreasing the frequency with which the same question is asked and enabling the person with dementia to appear calm and content. It is not realistic to expect to be able to eliminate repetitive questions.

- *Give cues about previous conversations.*

WHY ➔ If you frame the conversation to make allowances for their short-term memory loss, you may be able to have a conversation that is more satisfying to yourself. For example, if you ask, "What should we have for dinner tonight?", you may remember what you've eaten recently, but the person with dementia doesn't. If you say instead, "I'm tired of spaghetti, what else can we have for dinner?", you are more likely to get a useful response. By the way, figuring out what to eat for dinner is often frustrating, especially if you are not used to being the chief cook in the family. Making a list of all the possibilities together, and then using the list to plan the meals for the week and the necessary shopping, can provide structure to your day that will benefit both of you.

- ***Do not reason and argue***

WHY ➜ In order to reason or argue successfully, both participants in the conversation need to be able to remember what has been said previously during the argument, and what agreement may have been reached after a previous argument about the same topic. Anticipating the difficulty and gently guiding the person through what needs to be done may help. For example, trying to convince someone that they should not be driving, after they have lost their licence, will cause you to go back over topics that are very emotionally charged, such as their diagnosis and their relationship with the doctor. If you can, instead, acknowledge their grief over their loss and offer them sympathy, and then quickly make plans for the next outing the two of you can have together, it may help them think about a different topic that is not stressful to them.

- ***Do not expect that they can problem - solve.***

WHY ➜ Problem-solving requires keeping many factors in mind at the same time. People with severe short-term memory loss are able to keep only one thing in their mind at a time, and are not able to remember that, when they start thinking about the next thing. Simplifying a decision-making process by taking them through it one step at a time, or cutting out unnecessary steps, will help you to understand their wishes and needs.

Sometimes just doing what needs to be done without actually talking about it is more successful. For example, if you hold out their coat, the person with dementia may understand that they need to lift their arms into the sleeves. On the other hand, if you say, "You need a coat", they need to work at understanding your words and translating them into what actions they should perform, then remember what season it is and understand the implications for what they should wear, and then remember where their coat is kept and what it looks like. Once they get through that thought process slowly, they still have to remember to get the coat and put it on. Any distraction that interrupts them may mean that they forget to get their coat. Being mindful of eliminating the complexity, which requires a short-term memory for processing the information, provides kind and thoughtful assistance to a person with dementia.

Simplification of tasks and activities is necessary because dealing with short-term and long-term memory loss means the person with dementia is not able to understand the full context of a situation. Very often they perceive a context that is different from that context that you perceive - an altered reality. Supporting them, by helping them to maintain the understanding that they dwell in a place where they can be calm and stay secure both physically and emotionally, will help them to stay stable and functioning at their maximum capacity. If the person with dementia does not receive help in feeling emotionally secure, the altered reality they perceive may lead to them understanding that they are in an unsafe context and they may feel threatened, with the consequence that they may then act to defend themselves.

- *Do not expect them to remember*

WHY ➔ Sometimes it takes careful thought and problem-solving on your part to realize that expecting the person with dementia to do something requires the use of a memory process. Finishing their meal is one example. You may think that it is obvious if there is a plate of food in front of a person, they will keep eating until they are finished. However, other distractions may cause them to forget and they stop eating. When this becomes a problem, it takes time for you to learn what distracts them and how you can draw their attention back to their food without nagging or losing your temper. You may be able to listen to music or the radio through an earpiece to decrease your own boredom, if they would be distracted by it. Leaving the TV off and turning the ringer on the phone off for the duration of the meal may also save both of you aggravation.

- *Do not give corrections or scold for errors*

WHY ➔ Think of how irritated you become yourself if you are corrected or scolded. People with memory loss are making mistakes constantly. This may mean that they are constantly being scolded and corrected. Their irritation can build until they lose control of their temper.

- *Do not think they are uncooperative on purpose*

WHY ➔ Lack of cooperation usually stems from a lack of understanding and a fear of the situation. Simplifying the process, trying to figure out what is triggering their fear, delaying until they are calm, and maintaining a calm, unhurried and pleasant attitude will increase their ability to cooperate. Altering or eliminating activities will also be necessary as the disease progresses.

- *Do not think that they are pretending to forget*

WHY ➔ A person with dementia has no control over what they can and cannot remember, when they remember and when they do not, or whether their memory is sufficient to allow them to perform individual acts or functions. This is not a question of motivation or apathy. Inconsistency is part of the disease process. A person with dementia may be able to do something one day, but not the next. They may be able to remember who their younger daughter is, but not their older daughter. As you both go through your daily routines, you may have to alter how much help you give them, or how much or how little you need to say from day to day.

- *Do not act with impatience*

WHY ➔ As a person starts to develop dementia, they say and do things that do not make sense to others, things that seem to be unreasonable. They are starting to react differently because they are experiencing an altered reality, as compared to the reality that others around them understand. What makes sense to them, the way they understand their situation, is not the same as the common sense towards a situation as perceived by other people around them. This leads to many arguments. By the time a diagnosis is received, family members may have found themselves in a situation where impatience and argument are commonplace in their lives. This is not unusual and family members need to understand that rather than feeling guilty for their past impatience, they need to forgive themselves. Once the family knows it is dealing with dementia, however, it is important to try to undo the pattern of interacting with impatience and frequent arguments. Having to deal with your impatience is distracting and annoying for the person with dementia. This may affect their ability to function and their desire to converse or to be with you. Impatience and argument will interfere with getting through activities in a calm and pleasant atmosphere.

- *Use distraction to decrease distress*

WHY - People with severe short-term memory loss can usually concentrate on only one thing at a time. They have also lost the capacity to reason within themselves that a situation is not worrying and to calm themselves down. Guiding the conversation so that the one thing the person with dementia is thinking about is pleasant and non-threatening is helpful. For example, pointing out and commenting on various things you pass by as you are driving may displace repeated questions about where you are going and the anxiety about their destination.

6. B. Interaction that accommodates long-term memory loss

- *Talk about past events*

WHY ➔ In the Alzheimer pattern of memory loss, events that have happened in the past can still be remembered and talked about. Recent events have been erased and new memories are not usually made. The person with dementia cannot talk about things that they do not know. However, it is still important to both of you to converse in a pleasant social manner.

Some people become distressed because the person with dementia seems to dwell in the past. With a short-term memory loss, the present is simply not available to think about. The events that occupy the mind of a person with dementia are those to which they can access the memories - things that occurred in the past. They may or may not remember them accurately. Often events of the past that are emotionally difficult, such as wartime experiences, or times of family conflict, become dominant in the mind of the person with dementia. The carer may choose to become adept at leading the conversation away from emotionally painful topics.

- *Enter into their frame of reality*

WHY ➔ Looking for loved ones who have died is a normal part of memory loss due to dementia. If a person with dementia does not remember that their wife, husband, mother or father has died, they will naturally be concerned about them and look to see and talk to them. They are seeking the comfort of their company, especially because the experience of having dementia causes great stress. These were the people they turned to in the past for day to day activities and in times of need; since they don't remember they are gone they will naturally expect to be able to be with them. It will cause great distress to the person with dementia when they cannot find their loved one and they may feel that others are lying to them and trying to trick them, since that is the view from their reality. A carer cannot produce the missing loved one, but they can provide the needed comforting by understanding their reality and working to help the person with dementia regain a calm and stable view of their current situation.

Misidentification is also a normal part of memory loss in dementia. A person with dementia has lost the memory that a child has grown up and no longer remembers what their adult child looks like in the present. However, they may still remember that they have a child and be urgently concerned for that child's welfare. The person with dementia may also name current family members with the names of past, or older, family members because they retain only the names out of the past to use for people to whom they are currently feeling attachment and belonging.

Misidentification by people with dementia can cause great difficulty for others if the person with dementia is interpreting the relationship as romantic when their carer, family member or paid caregiver is not. This can happen when there is a relationship in which physical closeness is normal, such as that between a parent or grandparent and adult child or when a paid caregiver is giving intimate care. If the person with dementia does not remember who the other person is and what the relationship should be, the person with dementia will take cues from the interaction and make mistakes about what interaction is appropriate and what is not. This is not a situation that carers can or should accommodate. However, the carer must take great care to stay calm, or regain calmness themselves, in order to figure out how to control and manage the situation for the well-being of the person with dementia and everyone else involved.

- *Go with the flow of their unstructured past*

WHY ➔ The memories of the past that a person with dementia maintains may no longer be connected to the original time, or place, or person of the event. Refrain from arguing about what actually happened. The person with dementia has no control over their memory patterns. Arguing, reminding, or reorienting them does not help them change their mind about what happened, because their former memories are no longer available. The person with dementia cannot adapt to your need for them to have an accurate memory. You must be the one to adapt to the changes in them that result from disease.

We all have the feeling that we want other people to believe that what we say is the truth. This is one of the most difficult adjustments in being a carer for a person with dementia. We need to give up our need to be right, to be perceived as speaking the truth, in order to support an emotionally safe context for the person with dementia.

6. C. Accommodating Emotional and Procedural Memory

- *assist the person with dementia to remain calm, contented and stable*

WHY ➔ The experience of having dementia creates many negative emotions that cause great turmoil for the person with dementia and their family. Learning to create harmonious interactions is advisable in order to decrease stress and to increase the sense of security and safety of the person with dementia.

- *try to maintain a routine*

WHY ➔ The person with dementia is most likely to feel secure when they are doing the same things with the same person at the same time in the same place every day. When this happens, they are able to rely on their previous and new procedural memories to have a sense of being at home, belonging and being in a safe and predictable environment. When there are alterations in the routine, the person with dementia needs more engagement and emotional support by their carer in order to prevent them from becoming anxious.

- *try to make changes in daily routine slowly*

WHY ➔ A person with dementia relies on their remaining procedural memory to maintain whatever orientation to their life situation is possible. Drastic changes which happen quickly are more difficult for them to adjust to than a series of gradual small changes ("baby steps").

7. The Emotional Climate of the Carer

Nobody plans to have dementia, nor do they plan to be a carer for a family member with dementia. Dementia may occur when people are retired, and it interrupts and prevents them from carrying out the activities they had planned for their retirement years. A person who is working will have to stop working if they develop a disease causing dementia. If they have a spouse, that person may need to become the sole earner and the carer in the family. If a person's parent develops dementia, they may find themselves in the position of arranging care while they are trying to maintain the same level of performance in their job, care for their own family and continue to function in their community.

A carer inevitably needs to give up some of their activities in order to care for a person with dementia. The longer they deliver care, the more time and energy it takes as the condition of the person with dementia worsens. As time goes on, the carer must stop more and more of their previous activities.

While it is important to maintain a light-hearted and cheerful manner while interacting with the person with dementia, it is also vital to realistically assess the losses that both the person with dementia and yourself, as the carer, are experiencing. Acknowledging the losses allows you to understand your own emotional reactions and then to modify them in order to continue your care and whatever other activities you can accomplish.

Grief has been discussed and is inevitable as you mourn each disappearing memory and skill of the person with dementia, as well as the loss of your own former activities. Love and concern for a family member and pride in the care they are giving to them have carried many carers successfully through their journey with dementia. Many caregivers have said that keeping their sense of humour was very valuable to them.

Improvements in our medical care and sanitary conditions have enabled a large proportion of the population to survive into old age. However, now the number of people experiencing the diseases of old age has also increased. Changing lifestyles, nutritional inadequacies or excesses, and environmental toxins are also impacting on the incidence of dementia. Our health care systems have not yet caught up to this change and often people who need help coping with dementia in their families find the help offered inadequate to alleviate the stress and time demands they are experiencing.

Do not be afraid to advocate for help for yourself and for your family member with dementia to other members of the family, to health care agencies and to politicians. There is much room for improvement in the way we, as a society, support and care for people with dementia and their families.

Appendix. A Partial List of Emotions Commonly Affecting People with Dementia and their Carers

accepting	demeaned	humiliation	rejection
accepted	desire	humour	reluctant
accomplished	despair	ignored	remorseful
affection	determined	included	repulsion
agitated	disappointment	infatuated	resilience
alarmed	distressed	insulted	resistant
amused	doted on	isolated	respected
anguish	dreading	joy	restless
anger	elated	longing	sadness
annoyed	empathy	loss	safety
antagonistic	encouraged	lost	satisfied
anxious	endangered	love	shame
at ease	excited	loved	smart
attacked	excluded	melancholy	sorrow
attraction	expectant	mischievous	stressed
belonging	fearful	mistrustful	stupid
belligerent	flustered	motivated	suspicious
betrayal	fretful	needy	sympathy
calm	friendly	offended	terrified
cheerful	frustration	outrage	threatened
cherished	grateful	perturbed	uncertain
compassion	grief	playfulness	unfairness
concern	guilt	pleasure	unsafe
controlled	happiness	pride	upset
curious	hardiness	receptive	wary

About the Author

Jennifer Ghent-Fuller worked as a nurse in Canada for over twenty-five years, the last eleven as an educator and support counsellor for people with dementia and their families and other carers. Jennifer has a Bachelor of Arts from Queen's University (Kingston, Ontario), a Bachelor of Science in Nursing from the University of British Columbia (Vancouver, British Columbia), and a Master of Science in Nursing from the University of Western Ontario (London, Ontario). Jennifer has also worked as a volunteer in the fields of literacy and elder abuse prevention. She retired in 2011. In 2012, she published the book, "Thoughtful Dementia Care ™: Understanding the Dementia Experience."